51 Juice Recipe Heartburn Solutions:

Reduce and Prevent Heartburn by Drinking Delicious and Healthy Juices

By

Joe Correa CSN

COPYRIGHT

ACKNOWLEDGEMENTS

This book is dedicated to my friends and family that have had mild or serious illnesses so that you may find a solution and make the necessary changes in your life.

51 Juice Recipe Heartburn Solutions:

Reduce and Prevent Heartburn by Drinking Delicious and Healthy Juices

By

Joe Correa CSN

CONTENTS

ABOUT THE AUTHOR

After years of Research, I honestly believe in the positive effects that proper nutrition can have over the body and mind. My knowledge and experience has helped me live healthier throughout the years and which I have shared with family and friends. The more you know about eating and drinking healthier, the sooner you will want to change your life and eating habits.

Nutrition is a key part in the process of being healthy and living longer so get started today. The first step is the most important and the most significant.

INTRODUCTION

51 Juice Recipe Heartburn Solutions: Reduce and Prevent Heartburn by Drinking Delicious and Healthy Juices

By Joe Correa CSN

If you have ever felt heartburn, often described as a "fire in your chest", then you know how unpleasant this medical condition can be. It usually occurs after eating a heavy and greasy meal, smoking a lot, or drinking alcohol. This problem is more common than you think. About three billion people in the world suffer from this condition, at least once a week.

Modern lifestyles full of stress, poor diets and eating habits, unhealthy and processed foods, lots of caffeine, alcohol, and carbonated beverages have a harmful effect on our digestive tract and entire body.

In medical terms, heartburn can be described as acid indigestion. This burning sensation in the chest and/or upper abdomen appears due to regurgitation of gastric acid into the esophagus. Unlike the stomach that is lined with protective cells our esophagus doesn't have this protection. Naturally, when stomach acids and digestive juices reflux back, they cause serious inflammation and damage to gentle esophagus lining.

Preventing heartburn should be your number one priority in order to keep your digestive tract normal and healthy. Naturally, the best way to do this is to change your everyday eating habits. The most common heartburn triggers are:

- Alcohol

- Caffeine

- Over-the-counter medications

- Carbonated beverages

- Acidic foods and juice

- Smoking

These irritants increase the production of acid in the stomach and should definitely be avoided. However, there is much more you can do to heal the damage caused by years, even decades, of poor eating habits.

This collection of amazing juice recipes was designed to help you eat delicious and tasty ingredients, within a couple of minutes. Including these recipes into a healthy daily diet will give you an entirely new dimension of health benefits and flavors. These heartburn preventing recipes are based on fresh organic ingredients and aim to remove all those toxins and other chemicals often found in our organism.

Feel free to get creative and to add some additional ingredients if you like!

51 JUICE RECIPE HEARTBURN SOLUTIONS: REDUCE AND PREVENT HEARTBURN BY DRINKING DELICIOUS AND HEALTHY JUICES

1.   Spinach Cucumber Juice

Ingredients:

1 cup of fresh spinach, chopped

1 cup of cucumber, sliced

1 cup of fresh kale, chopped

1 cup of Swiss chard, torn

¼ tspof ginger, ground

1 oz of water

Preparation:

Combine spinach, kale, and Swiss chard in a large colander. Rinse under cold running water and slightly drain. Chop all into small pieces and set aside.

Wash the cucumber and cut into thin slices. Fill the measuring cup and reserve the rest in the refrigerator.

Now, combine spinach, kale, Swiss chard, and cucumber in a juicer and process until well juiced. Transfer to a serving glass and stir in the ginger and water.

Refrigerate for 10 minutes before serving.

Enjoy!

Nutrition information per serving: Kcal: 63, Protein: 9.9g, Carbs: 16.7g, Fats: 1.6g

2.   Watermelon Beet Juice

Ingredients:

1 cup of watermelon, cubed

1 whole beet, chopped

1 small Granny Smith's apple, cored

Preparation:

Cut the top of the watermelon. Cut lengthwise in half and then cut one large wedge. Peel it and cut into small cubes. Remove the seeds and fill the measuring cup. Wrap the rest in a plastic foil and refrigerate for later.

Wash and trim off the beet. Cut into bite-sized pieces and set aside.

Wash the apple and cut in half. Remove the core and cut into small pieces. Set aside.

Now, combine watermelon, beet, and apple in a juicer and process until well juiced. Transfer to a serving glass and refrigerate for 15 minutes before serving.

Garnish with mint and enjoy!

Nutrition information per serving: Kcal: 138, Protein: 2.8g, Carbs: 38.9g, Fats: 0.6g

3.   Banana Broccoli Juice

Ingredients:

1 large banana, chunked

2 cups of broccoli, chopped

1 cup of Romaine lettuce, shredded

2 oz of coconut water

Preparation:

Peel the banana and cut into small chunks. Set aside.

Wash the broccoli and trim off the outer wilted layers. Cut into small pieces and fill the measuring cup. Reserve the rest in the refrigerator.

Rinse the lettuce thoroughly under cold running water. Shred it and fill the measuring cup. Reserve the rest for later.

Now, combine banana, broccoli, and lettuce in a juicer and process until juiced. Transfer to a serving glass and stir in the coconut water.

Add some crushed ice and serve immediately.

Nutrition information per serving: Kcal: 153, Protein: 7.2g, Carbs: 44.7g, Fats: 1.3g

4.   Avocado Aloe Juice

Ingredients:

1 cup of avocado, cubed

1 cup of collard greens, chopped

1 cup of fresh mint, chopped

1 large Golden Delicious apple, cored

1 oz of aloe juice

Preparation:

Peel the avocado and cut into half. Remove the pit and cut into small cubes. Fill the measuring cup and reserve the rest for later.

Combine collard greens and mint in a colander. Wash thoroughly under cold running water and slightly drain. Chop all into small pieces and set aside.

Wash the apple and cut in half. Remove the core and cut into bite-sized pieces. Set aside.

Now, combine avocado, collard greens, mint, and apple in a juicer. Process until well juiced. Transfer to a serving glass and stir in the aloe juice.

Refrigerate for 10 minutes before serving.

Nutrition information per serving: Kcal: 318, Protein: 5.6g, Carbs: 47.7g, Fats: 22.7g

5. Fennel Ginger Juice

Ingredients:

1 medium-sized fennel bulb

1 small ginger knob, peeled

1 medium-sized carrot, sliced

1 large cabbage leaf, torn

Preparation:

Wash the fennel and trim off the green ends. Using a sharp paring knife, remove the outer layer. Cut into small pieces and set aside.

Peel the ginger knob and cut into small pieces. Set aside.

Wash and peel the carrot. Cut into thin slices and set aside.

Wash the cabbage leaf and torn with hands. Set aside.

Now, combine fennel, ginger, carrot, and cabbage in a juicer and process until juiced. Transfer to a serving glass and refrigerate before serving.

Enjoy!

Nutrition information per serving: Kcal: 72, Protein: 4g, Carbs: 25.9g, Fats: 0.7g

6.   Pepper Cauliflower Juice

Ingredients:

1 large red bell pepper, chopped

1 cup of cauliflower, chopped

1 cup of Brussels sprouts, halved

1 oz of water

Preparation:

Wash the bell pepper and cut lengthwise in half. Remove the seeds and the top stem. Cut into small pieces and set aside.

Trim off the outer leaves of a cauliflower. Wash it and cut into small pieces. Fill the measuring cup and reserve the rest in the refrigerator.

Wash the Brussels sprouts and trim off the wilted layers. Cut each in half and fill the measuring cup. Set aside.

Now, combine pepper, cauliflower, and Brussels sprouts in a juicer and process until juiced. Transfer to a serving glass and stir in the water.

Serve immediately.

Nutrition information per serving: Kcal: 106, Protein: 9.6g, Carbs: 30.9g, Fats: 1.3g

7.   Pumpkin Apple Juice

Ingredients:

1 cup of pumpkin, cubed

1 small green apple, cored

1 small pear, chopped

1 small ginger knob, peeled

1 oz of water

Preparation:

Peel the pumpkin and cut lengthwise in half. Scoop out the seeds and cut into small cubes. Fill the measuring cup and reserve the rest in the refrigerator.

Wash the apple and cut in half. Remove the core and cut into bite-sized pieces. Set aside.

Wash the pear and cut in half. Remove the core and cut into small chunks. Set aside.

Peel the ginger and cut into small pieces. Set aside.

Now, combine pumpkin, apple, pear, and ginger in a juicer and process until juiced. Transfer to a serving glass and stir in the water.

Add some ice and serve immediately.

Nutrition information per serving: Kcal: 167, Protein: 2.4g, Carbs: 50.7g, Fats: 0.6g

8.   Celery Asparagus Juice

Ingredients:

1 cup of celery, chopped

1 cup of asparagus, trimmed and chopped

1 large banana, peeled and chunked

1 small ginger knob, 1-inch thick

1 oz of water

Preparation:

Wash the celery stalks and cut into bite-sized pieces. Fill the measuring cup and reserve the rest for some other juice.

Wash the asparagus and trim off the woody ends. Cut into bite-sized pieces and set aside.

Peel the banana and cut into small chunks. Set aside.

Peel the ginger knob and chop it.

Now, combine celery, asparagus, banana, and ginger in a juicer and process until juiced. Transfer to a serving glass and stir in the water.

Add some crushed ice and serve immediately.

Nutrition information per serving: Kcal: 138, Protein: 5.3g, Carbs: 40.3g, Fats: 0.8g

9.   Cauliflower Carrot Juice

Ingredients:

1 cup of cauliflower, chopped

1 cup of carrots, sliced

1 cup of purple cabbage, chopped

1 cup of collard greens, chopped

Preparation:

Wash the cauliflower and trim off the outer leaves. Cut into bite-sized pieces and fill the measuring cup. Reserve the rest for later.

Wash and peel the carrots. Cut into thin slices and fill the measuring cup. Set aside.

Combine cabbage and collard greens in a colander. Wash thoroughly under cold running water and slightly drain. Chop into small pieces and set aside.

Now, combine cauliflower, carrots, cabbage, and collard greens in a juicer and process until juiced. Transfer to a serving glass and refrigerate for 10 minutes before serving.

Nutrition information per serving: Kcal: 138, Protein: 5.3g, Carbs: 40.3g, Fats: 0.8g

10.   Kale Banana Juice

Ingredients:

1 cup of fresh kale, chopped

1 large banana, peeled and chunked

1 small Granny Smith's apple, cored

1 cup of Brussels sprouts, halved

¼ tsp of ginger, ground

1 oz of coconut water

Preparation:

Wash the kale thoroughly under cold running water and slightly drain. Chop into small pieces and set aside.

Peel the banana and cut into small chunks. Set aside.

Wash the apple and cut in half. Remove the core and cut into bite-sized pieces. Set aside.

Wash the Brussels sprouts and remove the outer wilted layers. Cut each in half and set aside.

Now, combine kale, banana, apple, and Brussels sprouts in a juicer and process until juiced. Transfer to a serving glass and stir in the coconut water and ginger.

Add some ice and serve immediately.

Nutrition information per serving: Kcal: 223, Protein: 7.9g, Carbs: 64.4g, Fats: 1.6g

11.   Leek Potato Juice

Ingredients:

1 whole leek, chopped

1 cup of sweet potatoes, cubed

1 cup of turnip greens, torn

1 cup of cucumber, sliced

1 large carrot, sliced

¼ tsp of salt

1 oz of water

Preparation:

Wash the leek and cut into bite-sized pieces. Set aside.

Peel the potato and cut into small cubes. Fill the measuring cup and reserve the rest for later.

Place the turnip greens in a colander and rinse under running water. Slightly drain and torn with hands. Set aside.

Peel the cucumber and cut into thin slices. Fill the measuring cup and reserve the rest in the refrigerator.

Wash and peel the carrot. Cut into thin slices and set aside.

Now, combine leek, potato, turnip greens, cucumber, and carrot in a juicer and process until juiced. Transfer to a serving glass and stir in the salt and water.

Serve cold.

Nutrition information per serving: Kcal: 186, Protein: 5.3g, Carbs: 52.1g, Fats: 0.7g

12.   Cauliflower Kale Juice

Ingredients:

2 cups of cauliflower, chopped

1 cup of fresh kale, chopped

1 cup of Romaine lettuce, chopped

1 cup of fresh basil, chopped

1 cup of cucumber, sliced

Preparation:

Wash the cauliflower head and trim off the outer leaves. Wash and chop into bite-sized pieces. Fill the measuring cup and reserve the rest in the refrigerator.

Combine kale, lettuce, and basil in a large colander. Wash thoroughly under cold running water and slightly drain. Chop all into small pieces and set aside.

Wash the cucumber and cut into thin slices. Fill the measuring cup and reserve the rest for later. Set aside.

Now, combine cauliflower, kale, lettuce, basil, and cucumber in a juicer and process until juiced. Transfer to a serving glass and refrigerate for 10 minutes before serving.

Enjoy!

Nutrition information per serving: Kcal: 76, Protein: 8.6g, Carbs: 20.6g, Fats: 1.6g

13. Guava Pineapple Juice

Ingredients:

1 whole guava, chopped

1 cup of pineapple, chunked

1 cup of cucumber, sliced

1 cup of fresh mint, torn

1 oz of water

Preparation:

Wash and peel the guava fruit. Chop into bite-sized pieces and set aside.

Cut the top of the pineapple and peel it using a sharp paring knife. Peel it and cut into small pieces. Set aside.

Wash the cucumber and cut into thin slices. Fill the measuring cup and reserve the rest in the refrigerator.

Wash the mint and slightly drain. Torn with hands and set aside.

Now, combine guava, pineapple, cucumber, and mint in a juicer and process until juiced. Transfer to a serving glass and stir in the water.

Refrigerate for 10 minutes before serving.

Nutrition information per serving: Kcal: 115, Protein: 3.6g, Carbs: 35.2g, Fats: 1.1g

14.   Zucchini Pear Juice

Ingredients:

1 small zucchini, sliced

1 medium-sized pear, chopped

1 medium-sized banana, chunked

1 large strawberry, chopped

1 oz of water

Preparation:

Wash the zucchini and cut into small chunks. Set aside.

Wash the pear and cut in half. Remove the core and cut into bite-sized pieces. Set aside.

Peel the banana and cut into small chunks. Set aside.

Wash the strawberry and remove the stem. Cut into small pieces and set aside.

Now, combine zucchini, pear, banana, and strawberry in a juicer and process until juiced. Transfer to a serving glass and stir in the water.

Add some crushed ice and serve immediately.

Nutrition information per serving: Kcal: 191, Protein: 3.5g, Carbs: 59.1g, Fats: 1.1g

15.   Honeydew Mint Juice

Ingredients:

1 large wedge of honeydew melon, chopped

1 cup of fresh mint, chopped

1 cup of mustard greens, chopped

1 small Granny Smith's apple, cored

1 oz of water

Preparation:

Cut the melon in half. Cut one large wedge and peel the peel it. Cut into small pieces and set aside. Wrap the rest of the melon in a plastic foil and refrigerate for later.

Combine mint and mustard greens in a colander and wash thoroughly. Slightly drain and chop into small pieces. Set aside.

Wash the apple and cut lengthwise in half. Remove the core and cut into bite-sized pieces. Set aside.

Now, combine melon, mint, mustard greens and apple in a juicer and process until juiced.

Transfer to a serving glass and stir in the water. Refrigerate for 10 minutes before serving.

Nutrition information per serving: Kcal: 139, Protein: 4.1g, Carbs: 40.5g, Fats: 0.9g

16.   Brussels Sprout Pumpkin Juice

Ingredients:

2 cups of Brussels sprouts, halved

1 cup of pumpkin, cubed

2 large carrots, sliced

1 small ginger knob, peeled and chopped

1 oz of water

Preparation:

Wash the Brussels sprouts and trim off the outer wilted layers. Cut each sprout in half and set aside.

Cut the pumpkin in half and scoop out the seeds. For one cup, you'll need about one large wedge. Cut and peel. Chop into bite-sized pieces and fill the measuring cup. Wrap the rest of the pumpkin in a plastic foil and reserve in the refrigerator.

Wash and peel the carrots. Cut into thin slices and set aside.

Peel the ginger knob and chop it into small pieces. Set aside.

Now, combine Brussels sprouts, pumpkin, carrots, and ginger in a juicer and process until juiced. Transfer to a serving glass and stir in the water.

Add some ice and serve immediately.

Nutrition information per serving: Kcal: 127, Protein: 8.5g, Carbs: 38.2g, Fats: 1.1g

17.   Watermelon Cantaloupe Juice

Ingredients:

1 cup of watermelon, cubed

1 cup of cantaloupe, diced

1 small banana, chunked

¼ tsp of cinnamon, ground

Preparation:

Cut the watermelon lengthwise in half. For one cup, cut one large wedge. Peel and chop into small cubes. Remove the seeds and fill the measuring cup. Reserve the rest in the refrigerator.

Cut the cantaloupe in half and scoop out the seeds. Cut and peel two medium wedges. Fill the measuring cup and reserve the rest for later.

Peel the banana and cut into chunks. Set aside.

Now, combine watermelon, cantaloupe, and banana in a juicer and process until juiced. Transfer to a serving glass and stir in the cinnamon. Refrigerate for 10 minutes before serving.

Enjoy!

Nutrition information per serving: Kcal: 171, Protein: 3.4g, Carbs: 47.3g, Fats: 0.8g

18.   Potato Cabbage Juice

Ingredients:

1 cup of sweet potatoes, cubed

1 medium-sized artichoke, chopped

1 cup of cucumber, sliced

1 cup of green cabbage, chopped

Preparation:

Peel the sweet potato and cut into small cubes. Fill the measuring cup and reserve the rest for some other juice. Set aside.

Using a sharp paring knife, peel the artichoke and cut into bite-sized pieces. Set aside.

Wash the cucumber and cut into thin slices. fill the measuring cup and reserve the rest for later.

Wash the cabbage thoroughly under cold running water and torn with hands. Set aside.

Now, combine potato, artichoke, cucumber, and cabbage in a juicer and process until juiced. Transfer to a serving glass and refrigerate for 10 minutes before serving.

Enjoy!

Nutrition information per serving: Kcal: 150, Protein: 7.7g, Carbs: 47.3g, Fats: 0.4g

19.   Apple Ginger Juice

Ingredients:

1 small Granny Smith's apple, cored

1 small ginger knob, peeled and sliced

1 small pear, cored and chopped

1 small banana, peeled and chunked

1 cup of fresh spinach, chopped

Preparation:

Wash the apple and cut in half. Remove the core and cut into bite-sized pieces. Set aside.

Peel the ginger knob and chop into small pieces. Set aside.

Wash the pear and remove the core. Cut into small pieces and set aside.

Peel the banana and cut into small chunks. Set aside.

Wash the spinach thoroughly under cold running water. Slightly drain and chop into small pieces. Set aside.

Now, combine apple, ginger, pear, banana, and spinach in a juicer and process until juiced. Transfer to a serving glass and refrigerate for 10 minutes before serving.

Enjoy!

Nutrition information per serving: Kcal: 247, Protein: 1.7g, Carbs: 73.9g, Fats: 1.7g

20. Artichoke Broccoli Juice

Ingredients:

1 medium-sized artichoke, chopped

1 cup of fresh broccoli, chopped

1 cup of Swiss chard, chopped

1 cup of cucumber, sliced

1 oz of water

Preparation:

Trim off the outer leaves of the artichoke using a sharp paring knife. Wash it and cut into bite-sized pieces. Set aside.

Wash the broccoli and cut into small pieces. Fill the measuring cup and reserve the rest for later. Set aside.

Rinse the Swiss chard under cold running water. Slightly drain and chop into small pieces. Fill the measuring cup and reserve the rest in the refrigerator.

Wash the cucumber and cut into thin slices. Fill the measuring cup and reserve the rest in the refrigerator. Set aside.

Now, combine artichoke, broccoli, Swiss chard, and cucumber in a juicer and process until juiced. Transfer to a serving glass and stir in the water.

Refrigerate for 10 minutes before serving.

Nutrition information per serving: Kcal: 65, Protein: 7.7g, Carbs: 22.7g, Fats: 0.6g

21.   Spinach-Asparagus Juice

Ingredients:

1 cup of fresh spinach, chopped

1 medium-sized wedge of honeydew melon

1 cup of fresh wild asparagus, trimmed and chopped

¼ tsp of ginger, ground

Preparation:

Place the spinach in a colander and wash thoroughly under cold running water. Slightly drain and chop into small pieces. Fill the measuring cup and set aside. Reserve the rest in the refrigerator.

Cut the melon lengthwise in half. Scoop out the seeds and cut one medium-sized wedge. Peel it and cut into bite-sized pieces. Set aside.

Wash the asparagus and trim off the woody ends. Cut into bite-sized pieces and set aside.

Now, combine spinach, melon, and asparagus in a juicer and process until juiced. Transfer to a serving glass and stir in the ginger. Add some ice and serve immediately.

Nutrition information per serving: Kcal: 85, Protein: 9.6g, Carbs: 24.2g, Fats: 1.2g

22.   Celery Leek Juice

Ingredients:

2 cups of celery, chopped

1 whole leek, chopped

1 cup of cucumber, sliced

1 cup of fresh basil, chopped

Preparation:

Wash the celery and cut into bite-sized pieces. Fill the measuring cups and reserve the rest for later. Set aside.

Wash the leek and cut into small pieces. Set aside.

Wash the cucumber and cut into thin slices. Fill the measuring cup and reserve the rest for later. Set aside.

Wash the basil thoroughly under cold running water and slightly drain. Chop into small pieces and set aside.

Now, combine celery, leek, cucumber, and basil in a juicer and process until juiced. Transfer to a serving glass and refrigerate for 10 minutes.

Enjoy!

Nutrition information per serving: Kcal: 79, Protein: 3.8g, Carbs: 21.2g, Fats: 0.8g

23. Coconut Mango Juice

Ingredients:

1 cup of mango, chunked

1 large carrot, sliced

1 small Granny Smith's apple, cored and chopped

1 oz of coconut water

Preparation:

Peel the mango and cut into chunks. Fill the measuring cup and reserve the rest for later.

Wash and peel the carrot. Cut into bite-sized pieces and set aside.

Wash the apple and cut in half. Remove the core and cut into bite-sized pieces. Set aside.

Now, combine mango, carrot, and apple in a juicer and process until juiced. Transfer to a serving glass and stir in the coconut water. Add some crushed ice and serve immediately.

Enjoy!

Nutrition information per serving: Kcal: 179, Protein: 2.6g, Carbs: 51.2g, Fats:1.1g

24.   Squash Carrot Juice

Ingredients:

1 cup of butternut squash, cubed

4 baby carrots, sliced

1 cup of green cabbage, chopped

1 cup of cucumber, sliced

¼ tsp of turmeric, ground

Preparation:

Cut the butternut squash lengthwise in half. Scoop out the seeds and cut one large wedge. Peel and chop into small cubes. Wrap the rest of the squash in a plastic foil and place it in the refrigerator.

Wash and peel the carrots. Cut into thin slices and set aside.

Wash the cabbage thoroughly under cold running water. Chop into small pieces and fill the measuring cup. Reserve the rest for later.

Wash the cucumber and cut into thin slices. Fill the measuring cup and reserve the rest for later.

Now, combine squash, carrots, cabbage, and cucumber in a juicer and process until juiced. Transfer to a serving glass and stir in the turmeric.

Refrigerate for 15 minutes before serving.

Nutrition information per serving: Kcal: 108, Protein: 4.1g, Carbs: 35g, Fats: 0.6g

25.   Grape Pear Juice

Ingredients:

1 cup of green grapes

1 medium-sized pear, chopped

1 small zucchini, cut into bite-sized cubes

¼ tsp of cinnamon, ground

3 tbsp of coconut water

Preparation:

Wash the grapes and fill the measuring cup. Set aside.

Wash the pear and cut in half. Remove the core and cut into small pieces. Set aside.

Peel the zucchini and cut into bite-sized cubes. Set aside.

Now, combine grapes, pear, and zucchini in a juicer and process until juiced. Transfer to a serving glass and stir in the cinnamon and coconut water.

Add some crushed ice and serve immediately.

Enjoy!

Nutrition information per serving: Kcal: 153, Protein: 2.6 g, Carbs: 46.6g, Fats: 0.9g

26. Celery Banana Juice

Ingredients:

1 medium-sized banana, peeled and chunked

1 cup of celery, chopped

1 cup of watermelon, diced

1 oz of water

Preparation:

Peel the banana and cut into small chunks. Set aside.

Wash the celery and cut into bite-sized pieces. Fill the measuring cup and reserve the rest for later.

Cut the watermelon in half. For one cup, you'll need one large wedge. Peel and dice into small pieces. Remove the pits and fill the measuring cup. Wrap the rest of the melon in a plastic foil and refrigerate for later.

Now, combine banana, celery, and watermelon in a juicer and process until juiced. Transfer to a serving glass and stir in the water.

Add some ice and serve immediately.

Enjoy!

Nutrition information per serving: Kcal: 147, Protein: 2.9g, Carbs: 41.4g, Fats: 0.8g

27.   Cabbage Lettuce Juice

Ingredients:

1 cup of green cabbage, chopped

1 cup of Romaine lettuce, chopped

1 cup of broccoli, chopped

1 cup of cucumber, sliced

¼ tsp of salt

Preparation:

Combine cabbage and lettuce in a large colander. Wash thoroughly under cold running water and slightly drain. Chop into small pieces and set aside.

Wash the broccoli and trim off the white part. Cut into bite-sized pieces and fill the measuring cup. Set aside.

Wash the cucumber and cut into thin slices. Fill the measuring cup and reserve the rest in the refrigerator.

Now, combine cabbage, lettuce, broccoli, and cucumber in a juicer and process until well juiced. Transfer to a serving glass and stir in the salt.

Add some ice and serve immediately.

Nutrition information per serving: Kcal: 58, Protein: 5.7g, Carbs: 19.8g, Fats: 0.7g

28.   Peach Cantaloupe Juice

Ingredients:

3 medium-sized peaches, pitted and chopped

1 small wedge of cantaloupe

1 cup of pineapple, chunked

¼ tsp of cinnamon, ground

Preparation:

Wash the peaches and cut in half. Remove the pits and cut into bite-sized pieces. Set aside.

Cut the cantaloupe in half and scoop out the seeds. Cut and peel two medium wedges. Fill the measuring cup and reserve the rest for later.

Cut the top of the pineapple and peel it using a sharp paring knife. Peel it all and cut into small pieces. Fill the measuring cup and set aside.

Now, combine peaches, cantaloupe, and pineapple in a juicer and process until juiced. Transfer to a serving glass and stir in the cinnamon.

Refrigerate for 10 minutes before serving.

Nutrition information per serving: Kcal: 237, Protein: 5.4g, Carbs: 69.1g, Fats: 5.4g

29. Guava Carrot Juice

Ingredients:

1 whole guava, chopped

1 medium-sized carrot, sliced

1 cup of cucumber, sliced

1 medium-sized apple, cored and chopped

2 tbsp of coconut water

Preparation:

Wash the guava and cut into bite-sized pieces. Set aside.

Wash and peel the carrot. Cut into thin slices and set aside.

Wash the cucumber and cut into thin slices. Fill the measuring cup and reserve the rest for later.

Wash the apple and cut in half. Remove the core and cut into bite-sized pieces. Set aside.

Now, combine guava, carrot, cucumber, and apple in a juicer and process until juiced. Transfer to a serving glass and stir in the coconut water.

Add some ice and serve immediately.

Nutrition information per serving: Kcal: 128, Protein: 3.1g, Carbs: 38.3g, Fats: 1.1g

30.   Bean Turnip Juice

Ingredients:

1 cup of green beans, chopped

2 cups of turnip greens, chopped

1 small Granny Smith's apple, chopped

1 cup of cucumber, sliced

1 small ginger knob, peeled and chopped

Preparation:

Wash the beans and place them in a deep pot. Add 2 cups of water and bring it to a boil. Remove from the heat and drain well. Set aside to cool completely and the chop.

Wash the turnip greens thoroughly under cold running water. Chop into small pieces and set aside.

Wash the apple and cut in half. Remove the core and cut into bite-sized pieces. Set aside.

Wash the cucumber and cut into thin slices. Fill the measuring cup and reserve the rest in the refrigerator. Set aside.

Peel the ginger and cut into small pieces. Set aside.

Now, combine beans, turnip greens, apple, cucumber, and ginger in a juicer and process until juiced. Transfer to a serving glass and add few ice cubes.

Serve immediately.

Nutrition information per serving: Kcal: 122, Protein: 3.7g, Carbs: 34.2g, Fats: 0.8g

31.   Spinach Aloe Juice

Ingredients:

1 cup of fresh spinach, chopped

1 cup of fresh kale, chopped

1 cup of cucumber, sliced

1 cup of fennel, chopped

1 tbsp of aloe vera juice

Preparation:

Combine spinach and kale in a large colander. Wash thoroughly under cold running water and slightly drain. Chop into small pieces and set aside.

Wash the cucumber and cut into thin slices. Fill the measuring cup and reserve the rest for later. Set aside.

Wash the fennel and trim off the green ends. Using a sharp paring knife, remove the outer layer. Cut into small pieces and set aside.

Now, combine spinach, kale, cucumber, and fennel in a juicer and process until juiced. Transfer to a serving glass and stir in the aloe juice.

Refrigerate for 10 minutes before serving.

Nutrition information per serving: Kcal: 74, Protein: 10.3g, Carbs: 34.2g, Fats: 0.8g

32.   Banana Mint Juice

Ingredients:

2 large bananas, peeled and chunked

1 cup of fresh mint, chopped

1 small apple, cored

2 large strawberries, chopped

2 oz of water

Preparation:

Peel the bananas and cut into small chunks. Set aside.

Wash the mint and roughly chop it. Fill the measuring cup and set aside.

Wash the apple and cut in half. Remove the core and cut into bite-sized pieces. Set aside.

Wash the strawberries and remove the stem. Cut into bite-sized pieces and set aside.

Now, combine bananas, mint, apple, and strawberries in a juicer and process until juiced. Transfer to a serving glass and stir in the water.

Add some ice and serve immediately.

Nutrition information per serving: Kcal: 294, Protein: 4.5g, Carbs: 86.1g, Fats: 1.4g

33.   Chard Pineapple Juice

Ingredients:

2 cups of Swiss chard, chopped

1 cup of pineapple, chunked

1 cup of watermelon, diced

¼ tsp of ginger, ground

Preparation:

Wash the Swiss chard thoroughly under cold running water. Slightly drain and chop into small pieces. Set aside.

Cut the top of the pineapple and peel it using a sharp paring knife. Peel it all and cut into small pieces. Fill the measuring cup and set aside.

Cut the top of the watermelon. Cut lengthwise in half and then cut one large wedge. Peel it and cut into small cubes. Remove the seeds and fill the measuring cup. Wrap the rest in a plastic foil and refrigerate for later.

Now, combine Swiss chard, pineapple, and watermelon in a juicer and process until juiced. Transfer to a serving glass and stir in the ginger.

Add some ice and serve immediately.

Enjoy!

Nutrition information per serving: Kcal: 127, Protein: 3.1g, Carbs: 35.8g, Fats: 0.6g

34.   Sprout Cauliflower Juice

Ingredients:

2 cups of Brussels sprouts, halved

1 cup of cauliflower, chopped

1 cup of cucumber, sliced

1 cup of mustard greens, torn

1 oz of water

Preparation:

Wash the Brussels sprouts and trim off the wilted leaves. Cut each sprout in half and fill the measuring cup. Reserve the rest for later.

Trim off the outer leaves of the outer leaves of a cauliflower. Cut into bite-sized pieces and fill the measuring cup. Reserve the rest for later.

Wash the cucumber and cut into thin slices. Fill the measuring cup and reserve the rest in the refrigerator.

Wash the mustard greens thoroughly under cold running water. Slightly drain and chop into small pieces. Set aside.

Now, combine Brussels sprouts, cauliflower, cucumber, and mustard greens in a juicer and process until juiced. Transfer to a serving glass and stir in the water.

Enjoy!

Nutrition information per serving: Kcal: 91, Protein: 10.3g, Carbs: 27.5g, Fats: 1.1g

35.   Strawberry Watermelon Juice

Ingredients:

8 large strawberries, chopped

1 cup of watermelon, diced

1 cup of fresh mint, torn

1 small Granny Smith's apple, core and chopped

¼ tsp of cinnamon, ground

Preparation:

Wash the strawberries and remove the stems. Cut into bite-sized pieces and set aside.

Cut the top of the watermelon. Cut lengthwise in half and then cut one large wedge. Peel the wedge and cut into small cubes. Remove the seeds and fill the measuring cup. Wrap the rest in a plastic foil and refrigerate.

Wash the mint thoroughly and slightly drain. Torn with hands and set aside.

Wash the apple and cut in half. Remove the core and cut into bite-sized pieces. Set aside.

Now, combine strawberries, watermelon, mint, and apple in a juicer and process until juiced. Transfer to a serving glass and stir in the cinnamon.

Add some crushed ice and serve immediately.

Nutrition information per serving: Kcal: 154, Protein: 3.5g, Carbs: 45.8g, Fats: 1.1g

36.   Apricot Apple Juice

Ingredients:

3 whole apricots, chopped

1 small apple, chopped

1 medium-sized banana, sliced

1 medium-sized celery stalk, chopped

Preparation:

Wash the apricots and cut in half. Remove the pits and cut into bite-sized pieces. Set aside.

Wash the apple and cut in half. Remove the core and cut into bite-sized pieces. Set aside.

Peel the banana and cut into small chunks. Set aside.

Wash the celery stalk and cut into bite-sized pieces. Set aside.

Now, combine apricots, apple, banana, and celery in a juicer and process until juiced. Transfer to a serving glass and add some ice.

Serve immediately.

Nutrition information per serving: Kcal: 154, Protein: 3.5g, Carbs: 45.8g, Fats: 1.1g

37. Zucchini Parsnip Juice

Ingredients:

1 small zucchini, chopped

1 cup of parsnip, sliced

1 cup of watercress, chopped

1 cup of cucumber, sliced

Preparation:

Peel the zucchini and cut into thin slices. Set aside.

Wash the parsnip and trim off the green parts. slightly peel and cut into slices. Set side.

Wash the watercress thoroughly under cold running water. Drain and chop into small pieces. Set aside.

Wash the cucumber and cut into thin slices. Fill the measuring cup and reserve the rest for later. Set aside.

Now, combine zucchini, parsnip, watercress, and cucumber in a juicer and process until juiced. Transfer to a serving glass and stir in the water.

Add some ice and serve immediately.

Nutrition information per serving: Kcal: 99, Protein: 4.2g, Carbs: 29.9g, Fats: 0.9g

38.   Radish Leek Juice

Ingredients:

5 large radishes, chopped

2 whole leeks, chopped

2 cups of cucumber, sliced

2 cups of red leaf lettuce, shredded

1 cup of asparagus, trimmed

Preparation:

Wash the radishes and trim off the green parts. slightly peel and cut into thin slices. Set aside.

Wash the leeks and cut into bite-sized pieces. Set aside.

Wash the cucumber and cut into thin slices. Fill the measuring cups and reserve the rest in the refrigerator.

Wash the lettuce thoroughly under cold running water. Shred it and fill the measuring cups. Reserve the rest for later.

Wash the asparagus and trim off the woody ends. Cut into bite-sized pieces and set aside.

Now, combine radishes, leeks, cucumber, lettuce, and asparagus in a juicer and process until juiced. Transfer to a serving glass and add some crushed ice before serving.

Enjoy!

Nutrition information per serving: Kcal: 137, Protein: 7.3g, Carbs: 37g, Fats: 1g

39.   Honeydew Melon Avocado Juice

Ingredients:

1 large wedge of honeydew melon, chopped

1 cup of avocado, cubed

1 cup of mango, chopped

1 small ginger knob, sliced

1 oz of water

Preparation:

Cut the melon in half. Cut one large wedge and peel the peel it. Cut into small pieces and set aside. Wrap the rest of the melon in a plastic foil and refrigerate for later.

Peel the avocado and cut lengthwise in half. Remove the pit and cut into small cubes. Fill the measuring cup and reserve the rest in the refrigerator.

Peel the mango and chop into bite-sized pieces. Fill the measuring cup and reserve the rest in the refrigerator.

Peel the ginger knob and cut it in small pieces. Set aside.

Now, combine melon, avocado, mango, and ginger in a juicer and process until well juiced. Transfer to a serving glass and stir in the water.

Add some ice and serve immediately.

Enjoy!

Nutrition information per serving: Kcal: 347, Protein: 5.3g, Carbs: 53.1g, Fats: 22.8g

40.   Crookneck Squash Juice

Ingredients:

1 cup of crookneck squash, cubed

1 cup of pumpkin, chopped

1 cup of cucumber, sliced

¼ tsp of turmeric, ground

¼ tsp of salt

2 tbsp of water

Preparation:

Cut the squash lengthwise in half. Using a teaspoon, scoop out the seeds and clean it inside. Peel and cut into small cubes. Fill the measuring cup and wrap the rest in a plastic foil and refrigerate.

Peel the pumpkin and cut lengthwise in half. Scoop out the seeds and cut into small cubes. Fill the measuring cup and reserve the rest in the refrigerator.

Wash the cucumber and cut into thin slices. Fill the measuring cup and reserve the rest in the refrigerator.

Now, combine squash, pumpkin, and cucumber in a juicer and process until juiced. Transfer to a serving glass and stir in the turmeric, salt, and water.

Refrigerate for 10 minutes before serving.

Nutrition information per serving: Kcal: 73, Protein: 4.1g, Carbs: 19.3g, Fats: 0.9g

41.   Basil Avocado Juice

Ingredients:

1 cup of fresh basil, chopped

1 cup of avocado, cubed

1 small Granny Smith's apple, cored

1 small peach, chopped

1 oz of water

Preparation:

Wash the basil thoroughly under cold running water. Slightly drain and chop into small pieces. Set aside.

Peel the avocado and cut in half. Remove the pit and cut into small cubes. Fill the measuring cup and reserve the rest for later.

Wash the apple and cut lengthwise in half. Remove the core and cut into bite-sized pieces. Set aside.

Wash the peach and cut in half. Remove the pit and chop into small pieces. Set aside.

Now, combine basil, avocado, apple, and peach in a juicer and process until well juiced. Transfer to a serving glass and stir in the water.

Add some ice and serve immediately.

Enjoy!

Nutrition information per serving: Kcal: 315, Protein: 5.6g, Carbs: 45.4g, Fats: 22.7g

42.   Carrot Pineapple Juice

Ingredients:

1 large carrot, sliced

1 cup of pineapple, chunked

1 cup of blackberries

1 oz of water

Preparation:

Wash and peel the carrot. Cut into bite-sized pieces and set aside.

Using a sharp paring knife, cut the top of a pineapple and the peel it completely. Cut into small chunks and fill the measuring cup. Reserve the rest for later. Set aside.

Wash the blackberries using a colander. Slightly drain and set aside.

Now, combine carrot, pineapple, and blackberries in a juicer and process until juiced. Transfer to a serving glass and stir in the water.

Add some ice and serve immediately.

Nutrition information per serving: Kcal: 127, Protein: 3.6g, Carbs: 42.4g, Fats: 1.1g

43.   Potato Ginger Juice

Ingredients:

1 cup of sweet potatoes, chunked

1 ginger knob, sliced

1 large carrot, sliced

1 cup of cucumber, sliced

2 oz of water

Preparation:

Peel the potato and cut into small chunks. Fill the measuring cup and reserve the rest for later. Set aside.

Peel the ginger knob and cut into thin slices. Set aside.

Wash and peel the carrot. Cut into thin slices and set aside.

Wash the cucumber and cut into thin slices. Fill the measuring cup and reserve the rest for later.

Now, combine potato, ginger, carrot, and cucumber in a juicer and process until juiced transfer to a serving glass and stir in the water.

Nutrition information per serving: Kcal: 132, Protein: 3.2g, Carbs: 36.6g, Fats: 0.4g

44. Pear Raspberry Juice

Ingredients:

2 medium-sized pears, chopped

1 cup of cucumber, sliced

1 medium-sized banana, sliced

1 cup of raspberries

Preparation:

Wash the pear and cut in half. Remove the core and cut into bite-sized pieces. Set aside.

Wash the cucumber and cut into thin slices. Fill the measuring cup and reserve the rest for later.

Peel the banana and cut into small chunks. Set aside.

Wash the raspberries using a colander. Slightly drain and set aside.

Now, combine pear, cucumber, banana, and raspberries in a juicer and process until juiced. Transfer to a serving glass and add some crushed ice.

Serve immediately.

Nutrition information per serving: Kcal: 290, Protein: 4.4g, Carbs: 97.7g, Fats: 1.8g

45.   Papaya Mint Juice

Ingredients:

1 large papaya, chopped

1 cup of fresh mint, chopped

1 small Granny Smith's apple, cored

1 tbsp of coconut water

Preparation:

Peel the papaya and cut lengthwise in half. Scoop out the seeds and chop into small pieces. Set aside.

Wash the mint thoroughly under cold running water. Chop into small pieces and set aside.

Wash the apple and cut in half. Remove the core and cut into bite-sized pieces. Set aside.

Now, combine papaya, mint, and apple in a juicer and process until juiced. Transfer to a serving glass and stir in the coconut water.

Refrigerate for 10 minutes before serving.

Enjoy!

Nutrition information per serving: Kcal: 290, Protein: 4.4g, Carbs: 97.7g, Fats: 1.8g

46. Chamomile Juice

Ingredients:

1 tsp of chamomile tea

2 large carrots, sliced

1 cup of watermelon, diced

1 cup of cucumber, sliced

2 tbsp of hot water

¼ tsp of ginger, ground

Preparation:

Combine chamomile and hot water in a small cup or a bowl. Soak for 5 minutes. Set aside.

Wash and peel the carrots. Cut into thin slices and set aside.

Cut the top of the watermelon. Cut lengthwise in half and then cut one large wedge. Peel it and dice into small pieces. Remove the seeds and fill the measuring cup. Wrap the rest in a plastic foil and refrigerate for later.

Wash the cucumber and cut into thin slices. Fill the measuring cup and reserve the rest for later. Set aside.

Now, combine chamomile mixture, carrots, watermelon, and cucumber in a juicer and process until juiced.

Transfer to a serving glass and stir in the ginger. Refrigerate for 10 minutes before serving.

Enjoy!

Nutrition information per serving: Kcal: 96, Protein: 2.6g, Carbs: 27.2g, Fats: 0.6g

47.   Apple Aloe Juice

Ingredients:

1 small Granny Smith's apple, cored

1 tbsp of aloe juice

1 cup of cucumber, sliced

1 medium-sized banana, sliced

1 large celery stalk, chopped

Preparation:

Wash the apple and cut in half. Remove the core and cut into bite-sized pieces. Set aside.

Wash the cucumber and cut into thin slices. Fill the measuring cup and reserve the rest for later. Set aside.

Peel the banana and cut into chunks. Set aside.

Wash the celery stalk and chop into bite-sized pieces. Set aside.

Now, combine apple, cucumber, banana, and celery in a juicer. Process until juiced.

Transfer to a serving glass and stir in the aloe juice.

Add some crushed ice and serve immediately.

Nutrition information per serving: Kcal: 174, Protein: 2.7g, Carbs: 50.3g, Fats: 0.8g

48.   Avocado Zucchini Juice

Ingredients:

1 cup of avocado, cubed

1 medium-sized zucchini

1 whole leek, chopped

2 medium-sized asparagus spears

3 tbsp of water

Preparation:

Peel the avocado and cut lengthwise in half. Remove the core and cut into small cubes. Fill the measuring cup and reserve the rest in the refrigerator.

Peel the zucchini and cut into bite-sized pieces. Set aside.

Wash the leek and cut into small pieces. Set aside.

Now, combine avocado, zucchini, leek, and asparagus in a juicer and process until juiced. Transfer to a serving glass and stir in the water.

Refrigerate for 10 minutes before serving.

Enjoy!

Nutrition information per serving: Kcal: 277, Protein: 22.9g, Carbs: 32.7g, Fats: 22.9g

49.   Pineapple Mint Juice

Ingredients:

1 cup of pineapple, chunked

1 cup of fresh mint, torn

1 cup of watercress, chopped

1 cup of Romaine lettuce, torn

¼ tsp of ginger, ground

Preparation:

Cut the top of the pineapple and peel it using a sharp paring knife. Peel it and cut into small pieces. Set aside.

Combine watercress, mint, and lettuce in a large colander. Wash thoroughly under cold running water and torn into small pieces. Set aside.

Now, combine pineapple, mint, watercress, and lettuce in a juicer. Process until juiced.

Transfer to a serving glass and add some ice before serving.

Enjoy!

Nutrition information per serving: Kcal: 90, Protein: 3.2g, Carbs: 27.3g, Fats: 0.6g

50.   Melon Ginger Juice

Ingredients:

1 cup of watermelon, diced

1 medium-sized wedge of honeydew melon

1 small ginger knob, peeled and chopped

1 medium-sized carrot, sliced

1 small banana, chunked

Preparation:

Cut the top of the watermelon. Cut lengthwise in half and then cut one large wedge. Peel it and cut into small cubes. Remove the seeds and fill the measuring cup. Wrap the rest in a plastic foil and refrigerate for later.

Cut the melon in half. Cut one large wedge and peel the peel it. Cut into small pieces and set aside. Wrap the rest of the melon in a plastic foil and refrigerate for some other juice.

Peel the ginger and cut into small pieces. Set aside.

Wash and peel the carrot. Cut into thin slices and set aside.

Peel the banana and cut into chunks. Set aside.

Now, combine watermelon, honeydew melon, ginger, carrot, and banana in a juicer. Process until juiced.

Transfer to a serving glass and add some crushed ice before serving.

Enjoy!

Nutrition information per serving: Kcal: 188, Protein: 3.4g, Carbs: 52.8g, Fats: 0.9g

51.   Pear Cucumber Juice

Ingredients:

1 medium-sized pear, cored

1 cup of cucumber, sliced

1 cup of kale, torn

1 small green apple, cored

Preparation:

Wash the pear and cut lengthwise in half. Remove the core and cut into bite-sized pieces.

Wash the cucumber and cut into thin slices. Fill the measuring cup and reserve the rest for later. Set aside.

Wash the kale thoroughly under cold running water and slightly drain. Torn with hands and set aside.

Wash the apple and remove the core. Cut into small pieces and set aside.

Now, combine pear, cucumber, kale, and apple in a juicer and process until juiced. Transfer to a serving glass and add some ice before serving.

Enjoy!

Nutrition information per serving: Kcal: 177, Protein: 4.4g, Carbs: 54.5g, Fats: 1.2g

ADDITIONAL TITLES FROM THIS AUTHOR

70 Effective Meal Recipes to Prevent and Solve Being Overweight: Burn Fat Fast by Using Proper Dieting and Smart Nutrition

By Joe Correa CSN

48 Acne Solving Meal Recipes: The Fast and Natural Path to Fixing Your Acne Problems in Less Than 10 Days!

By Joe Correa CSN

41 Alzheimer's Preventing Meal Recipes: Reduce or Eliminate Your Alzheimer's Condition in 30 Days or Less!

By Joe Correa CSN

70 Effective Breast Cancer Meal Recipes: Prevent and Fight Breast Cancer with Smart Nutrition and Powerful Foods

By Joe Correa CSN

www.ingramcontent.com/pod-product-compliance
Lightning Source LLC
Chambersburg PA
CBHW030256030426
42336CB00009B/402